Strong from Within

**Fit mom wellness guide:
A Mother's Guide to Physical Resilience**

BY
EMILY HARLOW

Embracing Physical Resilience in Motherhood
Table of content:

Introduction

Embracing physical resilience becomes essential to handling the many joys and challenges that come with having a family during the parenting experience. The book "Strong from Within: A Mother's Guide to Physical Resilience" provides proof of a mother's ability to reinforce herself from the inside out as well as nurture others. Beyond the traditional narrative of sacrifice and tiredness, this book seeks to shed light on the transforming possibilities that physical resilience provides for mothers.

The introduction explores the fundamentals of physical resilience, presenting it as a force that is dynamic and transcends simple endurance. It investigates the idea that a resilient mother is one who flourishes, finding joy in the journey and strength in adversity, in addition to managing the pressures of everyday life. We will explore the mental and physical aspects of resilience as we go along, learning how a strong mentality and a healthy body serve as a resilient mother's foundation.

This guide fosters a sense of empowerment that comes from a strong, resilient core by encouraging moms to prioritize their well-being via real-life tales, professional insights, and helpful guidance. Mothers who embrace physical resilience might find a revitalized energy that improves their own lives and has a good impact on their families' well-being. Every mother is invited by this book to rediscover her power, embrace her resiliency, and set out on a path toward holistic wellbeing.

Chapter 1:
The Foundation of Strength - Building a Resilient Mindset

It is impossible to overestimate the importance of having a resilient mindset in the complex fabric of parenting, where demands are constant and problems are diverse. The foundation of enduring strength is having the mental toughness to get through the highs and lows of parenthood. In order to help moms on this life-changing journey, our investigation into "The Foundation of Strength" aims to disentangle the intricacies of developing a resilient attitude by offering advice, techniques, and uplifting stories.

The power of perspective:

The power of perspective is the foundation of a resilient attitude. The way that one views obstacles and failures has a big influence on mental toughness. Due to the abundance of obligations that mothers frequently face, worry and self-doubt can easily take over. However, moms can develop a mindset that flourishes in adversity by reinterpreting obstacles as chances for development and education. One of the most important steps in developing mental resilience is to change the emphasis from problems to solutions.

Accepting Modification and Flexibility:

Being a mother is a dynamic and always evolving experience. Resilient thinking is necessary to adjust to the changing requirements of children, from the restless nights of infancy through the turbulent adolescent years. Mothers can become more adaptable in the face of uncertainty by developing the skill of embracing change. Resilience in the ever-changing terrain of parenting is fostered by the capacity to modify expectations, remain receptive to novel approaches, and come up with innovative solutions.

Self-Care: The Foundation of Adaptability

A resilient attitude is centered on self-compassion. Mothers are typically driven by internalized pressure and cultural expectations to hold themselves to extraordinarily high standards. However, prioritizing self-compassion leads to the emergence of actual resilience. A foundation for enduring strength is laid by accepting that mistakes are a necessary part of the path and by being kind and understanding to oneself.

Gratitude's Transformative Power

Resilience requires the development of a positive mindset, and thankfulness is a powerful trigger for this change. Moms' mental resilience can be significantly impacted by taking the time to recognize their accomplishments, be grateful for their support network, and enjoy the little moments of happiness. Gratitude not only helps one to focus on what one has rather than what one lacks, but it also fosters a sense of strength and fulfillment that lays a strong basis for overcoming the difficulties of motherhood.

Anchoring the Present Moment with Mindfulness

Being fully present in the moment without passing judgment is the practice of mindfulness, which is a potent tool for developing a resilient attitude. Cultivating mindfulness provides a respite from the busy pace of motherhood, where multitasking and constant preparation are the norm. Mothers who practice mindfulness can reduce stress, improve emotional intelligence, and become more equipped to deal with unforeseen events. As mindfulness is incorporated into daily life, it builds resilience and encourages a composed, level-headed response to the responsibilities of parenting.

Having Reasonable Expectations

The sign of a resilient attitude is aiming for fair goals rather than perfection. Stress and feelings of inadequacy can result from having unrealistic expectations. Mothers frequently struggle with the pressure to perfectly balance their personal, professional, and family goals. Mothers can develop resilience by setting realistic goals and realizing that imperfections are a necessary part of the path. Mothers can cultivate a mindset that adjusts gracefully to the unpredictable nature of parenthood by accepting the ups and downs of daily living.

Social Support: Developing Resilience via Relationships

When it comes to developing a resilient mindset in motherhood, the adage "it takes a village" has a lot of meaning. Having social support is essential for fostering mental toughness. Creating a network of sympathetic family members, friends, and other mothers fosters a feeling of community. A mother's mental health can be greatly enhanced by talking to others about her experiences, asking for help, and realizing she is not the only one going through difficult times. Robust social networks function as a protective shield, offering psychological assistance during periods of strain and enhancing a mother's general adaptability.

Making Progress in Emotional Intelligence

Resilience is mostly based on emotional intelligence, which is the capacity to identify, comprehend, and control one's own emotions as well as those of others. Every day, mothers experience a range of emotions, including love and joy as well as irritation and tiredness. Mothers who have developed their emotional intelligence are better able to manage these feelings, react instead of responding, and keep their composure. Mothers can develop a resilient attitude that equips them to handle the emotional challenges of parenthood with grace by encouraging emotional awareness and management.

Taking Lessons from Failures and Setbacks

The capacity to recover from setbacks is what defines resilience, not the lack of them. One develops a resilient mindset by taking lessons from mistakes and disappointments. Mothers can treat setbacks as chances for growth rather of seeing them as insurmountable hurdles. Resilience is continuously developed via reflection on events, identification of lessons learned, and application of newly acquired wisdom in future undertakings. Every obstacle serves as a springboard for developing stronger mental toughness.

Self-Care's Significance in Mental Resilience

Self-care is essential to developing and maintaining a resilient mindset—it is not a luxury. In the effort to provide for their families, mothers frequently overlook their own health. But real resilience necessitates making self-care a priority. Sufficient sleep, consistent exercise, a healthy diet, and downtime are all critical elements of mental health. Mothers who understand the need of self-care as an investment in resilience are better equipped to handle the responsibilities of motherhood with strength and energy.

Developing an Attitude of Growth

Developing a progressive mentality instead of a fixed mindset is essential for developing a resilient perspective. Mothers who accept the notion that skills and intellect can be acquired via commitment and effort are more resilient in the face of adversity. A growth mindset promotes resilience in the face of adversity by promoting an optimistic outlook toward learning and progress. It cultivates the idea that difficulties are chances for development rather than insurmountable roadblocks.

Conclusion: The Constantly Changing Path of Resilience

To sum up, developing a resilient attitude throughout parenthood is a dynamic and always changing process. It includes accepting perspective, adjusting to change, self-compassion exercises, gratitude exercises, and mindfulness exercises. This transformational process involves several essential elements, such as establishing reasonable expectations, looking for social support, growing emotional intelligence, and learning from mistakes, emphasizing self-care, and cultivating a growth mindset.

Chapter 2:
Nourishing the Body: Nutrition for a Strong and Resilient Mother

The importance of nutrition is paramount in the hard terrain of motherhood, where the physical and mental health of the mother and child are connected. A mother's capacity to develop strength, resilience, and general well-being is closely correlated with her nutritional decisions, as "Nourishing the Body: Nutrition for a Strong and Resilient Mother" demonstrates. This thorough examination explores the fundamentals of nutrition and provides moms with expert guidance, doable solutions, and inspiring tactics to help them reach their health goals.

The Cornerstone of Health: Diets High in Nutrients

A nutrient-rich diet serves as the cornerstone of wellbeing for a strong and resilient mother. A mother's physical and emotional well-being is greatly aided by essential vitamins, minerals, and macronutrients. The body gets the nutrients it needs for energy, immunity, and general vitality when it eats a varied and balanced diet. Emphasis is placed on adopting a varied and healthful diet that serves as the foundation for a strong body, ranging from whole grains and lean proteins to a vibrant assortment of fruits and vegetables.

The Effects of Adequate Hydration

One of the most important things to remember when raising a child is to drink enough water. Water, however, is essential for both general health and physical toughness. Drinking enough water promotes healthy physical processes, facilitates digestion, and helps control body temperature. Staying hydrated is especially important during pregnancy and lactation, when the mother's body requires more fluids than the developing kid does. The investigation of water as a basic nutritional component emphasizes its significance in developing a robust and resilient mother.

Prenatal Nutrition: Establishing Hardiness Right Away

The process of becoming resilient starts even before a child is born. The health and development of the mother and the unborn child are greatly aided by proper diet throughout pregnancy. Important nutrients that support fetal development and establish the foundation for postpartum health during pregnancy include folic acid, iron, and omega-3 fatty acids. A thorough analysis of prenatal nutrition highlights the significance of a balanced diet, prenatal vitamins, and individualized treatment to guarantee the best possible health for mother and child.

Postpartum Nutrition: Healing and Adaptability

During the tremendous bodily changes that occur during the postpartum period, adequate nutrition is essential for recuperation and fortitude. In addition to restoring depleted minerals, addressing a new mother's nutritional needs also entails promoting lactation and maintaining hormonal equilibrium. The study of postpartum nutrition explores the importance of foods high in nutrients, consuming a sufficient amount of calories, and creating customized diet regimens to suit the specific requirements of new moms. The foundation for long-term physical resilience is laid by providing the body with care throughout this crucial stage.

Striking a Balance: Eating Well for Working Mothers

A typical challenge is juggling the obligations of parenthood with a dedication to a healthy diet. But even with a busy schedule, it is possible to keep your body strong and healthy. The study of nutrition for working mothers provides useful advice, time-efficient methods, and simple recipes that satisfy the dietary requirements of working mothers. With a focus on the significance of mindful eating and thoughtful meal preparation, this section offers busy moms a road map for implementing healthful choices into everyday life.

Superfoods and Powerhouses of Nutrition

Some foods are particularly notable for being nutritional powerhouses, providing a concentrated amount of vital elements. The benefits of including nutrient-dense foods like leafy greens, berries, nuts, and seeds in a mother's diet are examined in the discussion of superfoods. These superfoods offer anti-inflammatory, antioxidant, and other health advantages in addition to helping with physical resilience. Moms who are aware of the nutritional benefits of these superfoods are better equipped to make decisions that will strengthen and support their bodies.

Personalized Dietary Plans: A Comprehensive Method

Given that every woman is different and has different dietary requirements and preferences, the study of personalized nutrition is gaining importance. A comprehensive approach to nutrition takes into account a variety of aspects, including cultural preferences, dietary restrictions, age, and health status. Customizing dietary guidelines to meet the unique demands of every mother promotes self-determination and guarantees that dietary decisions are in line with personal objectives and situations. In order to develop a sustainable and successful nutrition plan, this section highlights the significance of consulting with healthcare providers or registered dietitians for tailored recommendations.

Emotional Consumption and Conscientious Eating

In the context of maternal nutrition, the complex link between emotions and eating behaviors is examined.

Stress, exhaustion, and other emotional variables are common causes of emotional eating, which can have negative effects on one's physical and mental health. The study of mindful nutrition explores methods for resolving emotional triggers, encouraging mindful eating, and developing a positive relationship with food. Mothers can develop better eating habits, strengthen their resilience, and create a healthier relationship with food by raising awareness and embracing mindful approaches to nutrition.

The Link between the Gut and the Brain: Eating Right for Mental Health

The gut-brain link, which emphasizes the complex interaction between the digestive system and mental health, is a growing field of research in nutritional science. The investigation of diet for mental toughness explores the influence of a balanced gut microbiota on mental health in general, mood control, and cognitive performance. Including prebiotics, probiotics, and a variety of meals high in fiber promotes a healthy gut flora, which helps maintain emotional stability and mental toughness. The importance of nutrition in fostering both physical and mental resilience is emphasized in this section.

Beyond Weight: Comprehensive Health Measures

Nutrition research for resilient and robust moms goes beyond conventional metrics like weight control. Rather, it promotes a comprehensive view of health that takes into account one's total vitality, energy levels, immune system, and mental clarity. By reorienting attention from outward appearances to interior health, mothers are more able to recognize the many advantages of healthy eating. Mothers can develop a resilient body that flourishes in the varied and dynamic terrain of motherhood by adopting holistic health strategies.

Sustainable Eating: Long-Term Well-Being and Adaptability

When investigating maternal nutrition, sustainability is a crucial factor to take into account. Adopting dietary practices that are not just nourishing for the body but also sustainable for the environment is essential to building long-term health and resilience. This section analyzes plant-based nutrition, talks about how dietary choices affect the environment, and recommends conscious eating. Mothers can nurture their own long-term health and resilience while also contributing to the well-being of future generations by adopting decisions that are in line with both personal health and global sustainability.

Conclusion:

Developing Nutritional Resilience to Empower Mothers

"Nourishing the Body: Nutrition for a Strong and Resilient Mother" concludes by emphasizing the significant influence that dietary decisions have on a mother's general wellbeing, emotional stability, and physical strength. Starting with the fundamentals of meals high in nutrients, exploring customized nutrition, and taking a comprehensive approach to health, this thorough investigation equips moms with information, tactics, and a fresh perspective on the critical role nutrition plays in their transition into parenthood.

The body needs nourishment for more reasons than just survival; it is a form of self-care, a pledge to resiliency, and a means of developing long-lasting strength. The decisions moms make about feeding their bodies go well beyond what's on the dinner table as they traverse the complex terrain of parenthood. They start to reflect a profound insight, which is that taking care of oneself is a prerequisite to taking care of others.

Mothers can protect their bodies against the physical strain of raising a family by adhering to the principles of a diverse, well-balanced diet, emphasizing water intake, and understanding the specific nutritional requirements at each stage of motherhood. Mothers are given useful skills to make educated decisions through the investigation of superfoods, customized nutrition, and mindful eating.

The focus on sustainable nutrition gives moms the chance to take care of their own immediate well-being as well as the health of the earth for future generations as motherhood progresses. It encourages consumption with awareness and the knowledge that decisions taken now have long-term effects on one's own health as well as the health of the environment.

"Nourishing the Body: Nutrition for a Strong and Resilient Mother" is ultimately a companion and guide on the life-changing path of parenthood. It honors the natural resilience that each mother possesses, realizing that through caring for their bodies, mothers are actively enhancing their own resilience rather than merely satisfying a biological need. A well-nourished body is the basis for enduring strength, steadfast resilience, and a meaningful journey through the complications and delights of motherhood. Decisions made in the area of nutrition become a potent statement of self-love.

Chapter 3:
From Bump to Fit: Prenatal Fitness and Preparation

The transition from pregnancy to motherhood is a life-changing experience that involves mental and physical changes as well as an increased sense of responsibility. In order to prepare expectant moms for the difficulties of labor and the postpartum phase, "From Bump to Fit: Prenatal Fitness and Preparation" delves into the critical function that prenatal exercise plays. This thorough manual explores the advantages of leading an active lifestyle while pregnant, as well as safety precautions and doable tactics to assist expectant moms in embracing physical fitness for a more comfortable pregnancy and easier adjustment to motherhood.

The Influence of Maternal Fitness

Prenatal fitness is a potent tool for boosting general well-being for both the mother and the developing baby; it is not simply about maintaining a specific level of physical activity. It has been demonstrated that frequent, moderate-intensity exercise during pregnancy offers many advantages. These include less risk of gestational diabetes, better weight control, improved mental and emotional wellness, and improved cardiovascular health. Prenatal fitness is shown to have a good effect on a mother's physical, emotional, and mental well-being in the investigation of its power.

Safety Advice: Choosing an Exercise Program During Pregnancy

Prenatal fitness has many advantages, but safety must always come first. Exercise should be done by expecting women while keeping in mind how their bodies are changing and the special requirements of pregnancy. This section highlights the significance of speaking with healthcare providers before starting any fitness program, answers frequently asked questions, and offers recommendations for safe exercise during each trimester. Safety factors also include workout selection, adaptations, and identifying warning indicators that may call for a stop or change in the fitness regimen.

Customizing Exercises for Each Trimester

Each stage of pregnancy has its own chances and challenges, making it a dynamic process. Workout regimens should be carefully designed to accommodate the changing needs of the body and the developing baby throughout each trimester. The manual examines workouts that are appropriate for every trimester and provides adjustments and alterations to take into account the mother's changing physical state. Through the customization of workouts to correspond with the unique obstacles and modifications associated with each trimester, expectant women can sustain a secure and efficient fitness regimen throughout their pregnancy.

Mind-Body Link: Prenatal Fitness's Emotional Advantages

In addition to its physiological benefits, prenatal fitness fosters the mind-body connection and provides emotional advantages that enhance the quality of a woman's pregnant experience. Exercise causes the release of endorphins, which lifts mood and reduces anxiety and tension. Prenatal fitness regimens that incorporate mindfulness and relaxation techniques further improve the mental health of pregnant mothers. This section delves into the significant influence of the mind-body connection on the emotional fortitude of soon-to-be moms, cultivating a feeling of serenity and empowerment.

Collaborating with Medical Experts

Working together with medical professionals who can offer individualized advice based on each pregnant mother's unique health profile is necessary for effective prenatal fitness. The manual places a strong emphasis on the necessity of speaking with midwives, obstetricians, or other medical professionals before beginning or altering a pregnant exercise program. Establishing a supporting rapport with medical specialists guarantees that training regimens are tailored to the mother's unique requirements, medical background, and pregnancy difficulties, promoting a secure and efficient approach to prenatal fitness.

Prenatal Exercise Types: A Comprehensive Perspective

Prenatal fitness refers to a range of physical activities that are tailored to the individual requirements and inclinations of pregnant women. The guide covers a wide range of possibilities, from low-impact exercises like swimming and walking to prenatal yoga and strength training. Prenatal exercise that takes a holistic approach guarantees a well-rounded fitness regimen that targets cardiovascular health, flexibility, strength, and balance. Prenatal workouts are flexible, so expectant mothers can select activities that suit their interests and fitness objectives.

Healthy Pelvic Floor: A Crucial Aspect

A vital component of pregnancy, labor, and the healing process after giving birth is the pelvic floor. Prenatal fitness is mostly dependent on the pelvic floor muscles being strong and in good condition. This section offers information on the anatomy of the pelvic floor, the value of pelvic floor exercises, and methods for enhancing pelvic floor health while pregnant. A more seamless labor experience and improved postpartum recovery can be achieved by placing an emphasis on pelvic floor awareness and adopting targeted exercises.

Hydration and Diet: Essential Elements of Prenatal Fitness

Adequate nutrition and hydration must be combined with physical activity throughout pregnancy. In order to ensure that the mother and the developing child receive the nutrients they require for optimum health, the handbook examines the critical role that appropriate diet plays in promoting prenatal fitness. Another important element that is emphasized is hydration, particularly during exercise. A healthy diet, maintaining hydration, and balancing energy requirements are all important for prenatal fitness and the health of the mother and unborn child.

Creating a Network of Support: Social Networks and Communities

Starting a prenatal fitness journey is not something you do alone. Creating a network of friends, partners, and other pregnant women fosters a sense of community and common experiences. The examination of social networks and community in prenatal fitness highlights the value of asking for support, exchanging knowledge, and creating a happy atmosphere. Participating in activities with encouraging friends, taking prenatal fitness courses, or joining online groups all foster a feeling of community that improves the overall experience of doing out during pregnancy.

Transitioning from Birth to the Fourth Trimester: Getting Ready

As a pregnancy develops into labor and delivery and beyond, attention turns to the postpartum period, which is commonly known as the "fourth trimester." The importance of getting ready for the mental and physical shifts that come with the postpartum phase is acknowledged in the guide. Techniques for managing postpartum recuperation, gradually reintroducing fitness, and modifying workout regimens in accordance with the body's changing requirements are examined. Prenatal training builds a strong, resilient body, which prepares the body for a more seamless postpartum transition and long-term wellbeing.

Final Thoughts: Encouraging Moms to Have a Safe Pregnancy Experience

To sum up, "From Bump to Fit: Prenatal Fitness and Preparation" is an all-inclusive guide for pregnant mothers who want to embrace exercise as an essential part of their pregnancy path. The handbook acknowledges the many advantages of prenatal fitness for mental and physical health as well as for preparing women for the demands of childbearing and parenthood. It also celebrates the transforming power of prenatal fitness.

This guide equips expectant mothers with the knowledge and skills to start a resilient and healthy pregnancy journey by addressing pelvic floor health, addressing nutrition and hydration, creating a support system, emphasizing the mind-body connection, navigating safety considerations, adjusting workouts to the trimesters, partnering with healthcare professionals, and planning for the postpartum transition.

In the end, "From Bump to Fit" emphasizes the notion that prenatal fitness is more than simply continuing an active lifestyle; it's a comprehensive strategy for self-care, a dedication to a healthier pregnancy, and a means of developing resilience and strength that go beyond the bump and into the life-changing experience of motherhood.

Chapter 4:
Postpartum Power: Restoring Physical Resilience After Birth

Known as the "fourth trimester," the postpartum period is a period of profound physical and mental transformation for new moms. "Postpartum Power: Restoring Physical Resilience After Birth" explores the self-care techniques, exercises, and necessary measures that help women rebuild their physical resilience after giving birth, highlighting the importance of postpartum recovery. With the help of this all-inclusive handbook, moms can face the postpartum journey with courage, strength, and a fresh commitment to their own wellbeing.

Comprehending the Postpartum Experience

Every mother's postpartum journey is distinct and personal, involving physical recuperation, emotional transitions, and the responsibilities of taking care of a newborn. An summary of the typical bodily changes that follow childbirth is given in this section, including hormonal changes, uterine contractions, and recuperation from labor and delivery. Comprehending the complexities of the postpartum phase paves the way for an all-encompassing strategy to rebuild physical resilience.

Accepting the Remedial Process

After giving birth, mending is a long process rather than a quick fix. Mothers are urged to approach the healing process with self-compassion and patience. The necessity of accepting and honoring the body's own healing schedule is covered throughout the guide. Every facet of the recovery process is examined, ranging from hormone changes to uterine involution and postpartum bleeding, to provide moms a thorough understanding of what to anticipate in the first few weeks and months following childbirth.

Pelvic Floor Rehabilitation: Bringing Your Core Back in Shape

Pelvic floor rehabilitation is a crucial component of postpartum healing. Targeted exercises are crucial for regaining the strength and functionality of the pelvic floor muscles, which are significantly strained during pregnancy and childbirth. This section outlines the benefits of pelvic floor exercises in preventing pelvic floor dysfunction and offers suggestions for incorporating them into a postpartum fitness program. Restoring core strength and fostering general physical resilience start with strengthening the pelvic floor.

Return to Exercise Gradually: Pay Attention to Your Body

Resuming exercise after giving birth is a process that needs to be done gradually, mindfully, and with great attention to the body's cues. The handbook places a strong emphasis on paying attention to your body, honoring its limitations, and easing back into physical activity. Starting with low-impact activities like walking and light stretching, moms may reacquaint themselves with their bodies and determine whether they're ready for more strenuous workouts. Resuming exercise gradually promotes mental health throughout the postpartum period in addition to physical recuperation.

Enhancing Muscle with Postpartum Activities

Exercises performed after giving birth are essential for regaining resilience and strength. Exercise regimens specifically designed to target pelvic floor strength, core stability, and general muscle toning aid in a slow and efficient recovery. A variety of postpartum activities are offered in this section, such as modified abdominal workouts, kegel exercises, moderate yoga positions, and pelvic tilts. These postpartum workouts are made to focus on specific muscle groups, improve flexibility, and promote general physical well-being.

Dietary Support for Healing After Childbirth

The foundation of postpartum recovery is proper diet, which offers vital nutrients for healing, vitality, and general well-being. In exploring the dietary requirements of new moms, the handbook highlights the significance of a well-balanced diet rich in nutrient-dense foods. Important considerations include drinking enough water, replacing important nutrients, and, if applicable, paying attention to the dietary requirements of breastfeeding. Eating healthful foods helps the body recuperate and maintains the physical toughness required to handle the rigors of parenting.

Optimal Mental and Emotional Health: A Comprehensive Perspective

There is a close relationship between mental and emotional health and physical resilience after birth. The manual promotes a comprehensive strategy for postpartum recuperation that gives mental health top priority. Techniques for handling postpartum mental disorders, getting support, and reducing stress are discussed. During the transforming postpartum time, mindfulness practices, relaxation techniques, and establishing emotional connections all lead to a positive mental outlook and enhanced overall resilience.

Sleep hygiene: An Essential Part of Recuperation

An important element of postpartum healing among the demands of caring for a newborn is establishing regular sleep patterns. Resilience in general, emotional health and physical recovery all depend on getting enough sleep. This section offers information on good sleep hygiene, such as setting up a sleeping environment that is conducive to rest, developing a regular sleep schedule, and handling sleep difficulties when caring for a newborn. Making enough time for a good night's sleep encourages the body's natural healing processes and improves recovery after giving birth.

Collaborating with Medical Experts

Working together with medical professionals is crucial in the postpartum phase. Frequent check-ups with midwives, obstetricians, or other medical professionals guarantee that any postpartum issues or problems are dealt with right away. The handbook places a strong emphasis on the value of being transparent with medical experts, getting advice on postpartum fitness regimens, and resolving any potential mental or physical difficulties. Developing a cooperative relationship with medical professionals is a crucial component of a thorough and knowledgeable postpartum recovery strategy.

Self-Care Routines: Taking Care of Mother

A crucial component of postpartum healing is self-care, which cannot be compromised in the midst of caring for a newborn. The manual covers self-care routines that put the mother's health first, such as mindfulness exercises, relaxation methods, and joyful and fulfilling pursuits. Establishing a self-care regimen eases stress, builds emotional fortitude, and enhances the postpartum experience. Maintaining the mother's physical and mental well-being is crucial for her overall wellbeing as well as for building a strong foundation for the family as a whole.

Developing Relationships with Other Mothers to Create a Community of Support

As the postpartum experience can be lonely, making connections with other mothers offers a vital network of support. Mothers are urged in this section to look for community through social media, online forums, or local support organizations. Creating a supportive network of fellow mothers, exchanging advice, and sharing experiences all help to foster understanding and comradery. Making connections with other moms creates a community of support where common struggles are greeted with compassion and group knowledge strengthens each mother's ability to withstand the specific challenges she faces after giving birth.

Accepting the Changing Path of Parenthood

To sum up,

"Postpartum Power: Restoring Physical Resilience after Birth"

is a useful manual for moms navigating the revolutionary time after giving birth. This extensive resource enables moms to regain their physical resilience after giving birth, from comprehending the healing process and pelvic floor rehabilitation to gradually returning to exercise, strengthening with postpartum exercises, and emphasizing mental, emotional, and physical well-being.

Mothers can successfully manage the joys and challenges of the postpartum journey by adopting a holistic strategy that includes self-care rituals, networking with other mothers, working in conjunction with healthcare experts, and placing a high priority on nutrition and good sleep hygiene. "Postpartum Power" acknowledges that building physical resilience following childbirth is a journey that calls for self-compassion, endurance, and a dedication to supporting the mother's physical and mental well-being rather than a one-size-fits-all approach.

Chapter 5:
Balancing Act: Juggling Motherhood and Fitness

Many moms face a complex road of juggling the obligations of motherhood with a dedication to fitness, frequently finding themselves in a delicate and dynamic balancing act. The book "Balancing Act: Juggling Motherhood and Fitness" examines the benefits and drawbacks of fitting a fitness regimen into a mother's hectic schedule. This thorough manual explores useful techniques, mental adjustments, and powerful ideas to assist moms in finding a healthy balance between taking care of their physical health and carrying out their responsibilities as caretakers.

The Motherhood Reality

Being a mother is a complex web of happiness, contentment, and occasionally, enormous responsibility. Moms have never-ending demands on their time and energy, from tending to home duties to feedings at night. The first section of the guide acknowledges the realities of motherhood, stressing the variety of obstacles that mothers encounter and the significance of adopting a flexible and realistic approach to fitness within the framework of their particular situation.

The Value of Making Self-Care a Priority

Mothers tend to put their own needs last when taking care of others. The manual places a strong emphasis on self-care and presents it as the key to successfully balancing parenthood and fitness. Making self-care a priority is essential for maintaining one's physical and mental health, not a luxury. The idea of self-care as an investment in one's resilience, health, and general capacity to meet the demands of motherhood with vigor and grace is examined in this section.

Changing Perceptions: Redefining Mothers' Fitness

It frequently takes a mental adjustment to successfully combine parenthood and exercise. Moms are urged by the guide to redefine fitness according to their stage of life at the time. Moms are encouraged to adopt a holistic perspective of fitness that includes a variety of physical activities, such as daily movements and activities with their children, as opposed to conforming to conventional ideals. Through mental transformation, moms can alleviate the burden of impractical demands and establish a long-term strategy for physical well-being.

Fitting Exercise into Everyday Activities

Integrating physical activity into everyday activities is one of the most important tactics for striking a balance between motherhood and health. This section offers helpful advice and imaginative suggestions for integrating exercise into moms' daily routines. The book covers everything from short at-home workouts to including kids in fitness pursuits, offering ideas for integrating fitness into everyday life in a fun and realistic way. Time limits and unpredictability are obstacles that mothers can overcome by incorporating exercise into their lives in a seamless manner.

Prioritization and Time Management

Managing your time well is essential when balancing mom duties with a fitness regimen. The manual provides information on setting priorities, time-blocking tactics, and realistic timetables that include time set aside for fitness-related activities. Mothers may make time for self-care and fitness by setting priorities and managing their time well. This will help these activities become essential parts of their everyday routines.

Including the Family: Creating a Shared Experience with Fitness

Mothers are urged to include their families in the fitness journey rather than seeing it as a solo endeavor. In addition to strengthening family ties, making exercise a shared activity gives moms a chance to set an example of healthy behavior for their kids. The book looks at family-friendly workouts that everyone can do, like entertaining workouts and group walks, to create a welcoming environment. Mothers who involve their family can build a network of support that helps them on their fitness quest.

Getting Used to Life Shifts: The Changing Motherhood Seasons

The journey of motherhood is characterized by many seasons, each of which offers unique chances and challenges. The significance of modifying exercise regimens to account for life transitions, including pregnancy, the postpartum phase, and a child's developmental phases, is discussed in this section. Mothers who adapt their fitness strategies to the various seasons can be resilient and flexible in navigating the ever-changing nature of parenthood.

Moving With Awareness: Promoting Presence in Exercise

Developing an awareness of the present moment while exercising is known as mindful movement. The concept of mindful fitness is introduced throughout the handbook, with a focus on the advantages of exercising while completely present. Exercises that involve mindful movement are more effective and also help with stress management and mental health. It is recommended that mothers adopt a mindful attitude to physical activity, cultivating a sense of awareness and awareness between their bodies and minds.

Getting Rid of Guilt: Crossing Emotional Obstacles
One of the most frequent mental obstacles women encounter while trying to put their own needs first is guilt. The manual offers techniques to get past the emotional barrier of guilt related to making time for fitness. Mothers can manage and overcome shame by redefining fitness as a crucial component of self-care and highlighting the benefits for both physical and mental health. This opens the door for a more empowered attitude to their well-being.

Seeking Assistance: Establishing a Mothers' Community
Having the support of a community can frequently make juggling parenting and exercise simpler. The significance of getting help from other mothers who have comparable difficulties and aspirations is discussed in this section. A sense of camaraderie can be fostered through joining exercise groups, taking part in online communities, or creating local networks. By creating a community of mothers, people can encourage one another, share experiences, and trade advice on how to effectively manage the juggling act.

Accepting Your Flaws: It's a Process, Not a Finish
Ultimately, the manual exhorts moms to accept their flaws and see the process of striking a balance between parenting and fitness as a continuous and ever-changing one. Mothers are advised to recognize failures, praise accomplishments, and modify their strategy as necessary, as opposed to aiming for perfection. The focus is on cultivating an optimistic and caring mindset that acknowledges the trip as a dynamic process full of learning, development, and self-discovery.

Final Thought: Succeeding in the Balancing Act
To sum up, "Balancing Act: Juggling Motherhood and Fitness" is a helpful guide for moms who must balance

taking care of their families with putting their personal health and fitness first. Mothers can thrive in the balancing act by accepting the realities of motherhood, making self-care a priority, changing perspectives, incorporating fitness into daily routines, managing time well, involving the family, adjusting to life transitions, embracing mindful movement, overcoming guilt, seeking support, and embracing imperfections.

The guide acknowledges that there is no one-size-fits-all method and that every person's journey toward motherhood and fitness is different. Rather, it empowers moms to choose their own routes, discovering happiness and satisfaction in the balanced fusion of physical health with the wonderful but hard job of motherhood. The delicate balancing act becomes a monument to the fortitude, tenacity, and dedication of moms who perform this difficult dance with elegance and resolve.

Chapter 6:
Core Connections: Strengthening the Foundation of Physical Resilience

Often called the body's powerhouse, the core is essential to overall health, stability, and physical resilience. The importance of a robust and well-conditioned core in promoting numerous facets of physical health is examined in "Core Connections: Strengthening the Foundation of Physical Resilience". This in-depth manual explores the architecture of the core, the advantages of having a strong core, and doable methods for fortifying this vital part of the body.

The Anatomy of the Core

Beyond the widely known abdominal muscles, the core contains a complex system of muscles. It consists of the diaphragm, pelvic floor muscles, rectus abdominis, obliques, transverse abdominis, and several muscles in the lower back and spine. Gaining an understanding of the structure of the core is crucial to creating focused and efficient plans for building strength in this interrelated system of muscles.

The Body's Powerhouse: The Core

The body's powerhouse, the core offers support, balance, and stability for both regular activities and vigorous motions. A strong core is essential for any activity, including lifting a child, reaching, and exercising. The stabilizing role of the core, its ability to transmit power and energy between the upper and lower bodies, and its role as the basis for functional movement patterns are all covered in this section.

Advantages of a Firm Core

There are several advantages to a well-conditioned core that go beyond appearance. The many benefits of having a strong core are discussed in this guide, which includes better posture, increased strength overall, improved balance and coordination, and a decreased chance of injury. Furthermore, improved spinal alignment, which reduces back discomfort and promotes ideal body mechanics, is facilitated by a strong core. Comprehending the all-encompassing advantages emphasizes how crucial it is to give core strength top priority in order to achieve total physical resilience.

Exercises for Building Core Strength: A Holistic Perspective

Starting a core strengthening journey requires a comprehensive strategy that focuses on different muscle groups inside the core complex. A variety of core-strengthening exercises are introduced in the guide, such as functional motions, stability exercises, and classic abdominal workouts. These exercises improve balance and general strength by using the core in a variety of planes of motion. A complete and efficient strengthening process is ensured by a well-rounded core routine, which takes care of the entire core complex.

Activation of the Core in Daily Life

In addition to specific workout regimens, the manual highlights the value of core activation in daily life. Maintaining the growth of core strength is facilitated by using the core during routine tasks like lifting, sitting, and standing. There are helpful hints for integrating core activation into everyday activities that will help raise awareness of the core's function in preserving alignment and stability during a variety of movements.

Posture and Core Resilience

Maintaining proper posture is essential to core resilience, and posture and core strength are closely related concepts. The connection between ideal posture and a robust core is examined in this section. There are core-strengthening exercises that target postural muscles directly, and advice on how to maintain good alignment during regular activities is provided. In addition to making one look better, good posture is essential for preventing musculoskeletal problems and fostering long-term core resilience.

Fundamental Training for Particular Objectives

Because core training is so adaptable, people can customize their routines to meet particular objectives. The guide offers guidance on tailoring core training for various goals, such as improving sports performance, reducing back pain, or promoting general well-being. We discuss goal-specific core exercises, adaptations, and progressions so that people can customize their core training to meet their own requirements and goals.

Core Stability During and After Pregnancy

Pregnancy and the postpartum phase present special chances and challenges to develop core strength. The significance of preserving core strength throughout pregnancy is discussed in this section in order to support the changing body and get ready for childbirth. Postpartum core workouts address the effects of pregnancy on the pelvic floor and abdominal muscles, promoting a progressive and targeted recovery process. In order to promote a secure and efficient method of preserving core resilience, strategies for customizing core exercises to the various phases of pregnancy and postpartum recuperation are described.

Mind-Body Link: Fundamental Awareness

A strong mind-body connection is essential for core training to be effective. The manual delves into the idea of "core awareness," stressing the importance of mindfulness in contracting and strengthening the abdominal muscles.

During core exercises, mindful movement practices, breathwork, and visualization techniques are introduced to improve the mind-body connection. People can maximize the benefits of their core training and foster a closer relationship with their body's powerhouse by developing awareness.

Gradual Core Exercise: Developing Strength and Endurance

In order to gradually increase strength and endurance, progressive core training entails progressively upping the complexity and intensity of workouts. The manual describes the fundamentals of progressive core training, which include adding obstacles like resistance and instability, varying up the exercises, and gradually increasing the amount of load. In order to avoid plateaus in the development of core strength, a progressive strategy guarantees ongoing adaptation and improvement.

Whole Health: Fundamental Fortitude Beyond Appearances

The article notes that while a toned midsection is frequently an obvious result of core training, core resilience has several advantages that go well beyond appearance. It is believed that core strength is essential to holistic health since it promotes injury prevention, effective movement, and general physical well-being. People are more inclined to consider core training as a crucial component of their journey toward health and fitness when they understand the wider implications of having a resilient core.

Essential Upkeep for Extended Health

Retaining core strength requires a lifetime commitment to resilience and long-term health. This section offers advice on core maintenance techniques, such as correcting imbalances, tailoring workouts to specific requirements and objectives, and adding frequent core exercises to fitness regimens. By considering core maintenance as a continuous process, people can build a strong and long-lasting basis for their physical health.

Closing: Strengthening Fundamental Resilience

To sum up, "Core Connections: Strengthening the Foundation of Physical Resilience" is an all-inclusive manual for people who want to improve their general health and core strength. People can strengthen their core resilience by learning about the anatomy of the core, appreciating the advantages of having a strong core, embracing progressive core training, recognizing the holistic health benefits, integrating core activation into daily life, stressing posture and alignment, customizing core training to specific goals, addressing core strength during pregnancy and postpartum, and developing a mind-body connection.

The handbook highlights the various advantages of having a robust and strong core, stressing that having a strong core is essential to maintaining an active and healthy lifestyle in addition to helping one's midsection look toned. Through developing a more profound relationship with the body's powerhouse, people can build a foundation of physical resilience that improves their quality of life in general.

Chapter 7:
Fit and Fun: Incorporating Playful Activities for Mother-Child Bonding

Being a mother is not just about providing care and nurturing; it's also about having fun and experiencing happy times with your family. In order to promote physical health and build the link between mothers and their children, it is important to incorporate playful activities into everyday routines. This is explored in the book "Fit and Fun: Incorporating Playful Activities for Mother-Child Bonding". This all-inclusive manual explores fun and inventive methods to incorporate fitness into family activities, creating an environment that is good for the body and the parent-child bond. Playful Activities' Power

Playful activities are beneficial for bonding, communication, and the general wellbeing of moms and their children. They are not merely for amusement. The advantages of include play in everyday activities are discussed in this section, with special attention on how play affects cognitive, emotional, and physical development. Playful activities have far more benefits than just being enjoyable; they can improve mood, reduce stress, foster creativity, and improve communication skills.

Adapting Activities to Development and Age

The handbook acknowledges that children's needs and skills vary depending on their age. Ensuring that the activities are age and developmental-appropriate guarantees that the child will benefit from and enjoy them. Age-appropriate activities create a good and encouraging atmosphere for mother-child bonding, whether you play interactive games with a toddler or take part in more structured sports with older kids.

Innovative Ideas for Indoor Play

Playing indoors can be just as exciting and lively as playing outside. The handbook offers imaginative and imaginative indoor play activities that encourage physical exercise. Regardless of the weather or available space, indoor play activities provide mothers a variety of possibilities to engage with their children in an active and entertaining way. These activities range from obstacle courses and dance parties to scavenger hunts and yoga sessions.

Outdoor Experiences to Promote Active Bonding

Engaging in outdoor activities allows mothers and their children to actively bond while enjoying the fresh air and natural surroundings. The book looks at outdoor experiences that blend the beauty of nature with physical health. Mothers and kids may interact, discover, and move in the great outdoors through activities like biking, hiking, and environmental treasure hunts. In addition to improving physical health, outdoor experiences help people make lifelong memories in a fascinating and natural setting.

Movement & Dance: Moving Together

Engaging in dance and movement activities can be an enjoyable means of improving physical health and coordination, in addition to being fun. Mothers and kids can groove together with the introduction of interactive dance parties, movement-based games, and dance routines in the guide. Dancing, with its rhythmic excitement, creates a sense of connection and shared energy, whether one is dancing to a set routine or impromptu dance-offs.

Exercise Difficulties: Friendly Rivalry

Introducing healthy competitiveness and enthusiasm through friendly fitness challenges enhances mother-child attachment. Age-appropriate fitness tasks that promote motivation, teamwork, and a sense of accomplishment are recommended by the handbook. Fitness challenges, such as putting up miniature obstacle courses, hosting friendly races, or taking part in sports drills, encourage physical exercise while fostering a supportive and encouraging environment that fosters relationships between moms and their children.

Including Educational Components

Engaging in playful activities can be a great way to include educational components in the bonding process. The handbook looks at exercises that combine academic ideas with physical conditioning. Mothers can employ playful activities to improve their child's learning while having fun and memorable experiences together. Examples of these activities include combining math and counting into games and using outdoor trips to explore science and nature.

Water Play for revitalizing Relationships

Playing in the water adds a revitalizing and lively touch to mother-child bonding activities. The guide offers ideas for integrating water play into workout regimens, whether at the pool, beach, or even in the backyard with water games. In addition to providing a fun and interesting method to stay active, swimming, water aerobics, and activities with a water theme foster a special and unforgettable setting where mothers and kids can bond.

Yoga and Quiet Times

For mothers and their children, yoga and other mindful practices offer a soothing and centering experience. Using stretches, yoga positions, and mindfulness exercises, the book caters to children's fun temperament. Including yoga into quality time with loved ones improves balance and flexibility while also encouraging awareness and relaxation. A comprehensive approach to fitness and well-being is made possible by incorporating times for introspection and silence into enjoyable activities.

Exercises with Partners for Joint Efforts

Exercises with a partner foster a culture of cooperation and support. The manual presents activities and routines that moms can carry out with their kids to promote encouragement and teamwork. Partner workouts, whether they involve bodyweight exercises, stretches, or basic strength-building activities, improve the mother-child relationship's sense of teamwork and mutual success.

Using Movement to Tell Stories

Mother-child bonding takes on a narrative dimension when movement activities are integrated with storytelling. The manual recommends mixing narratives, fictional characters, and creative situations into movement-based exercises. Storytelling through movement turns physical activity into a creative and storytelling journey that fortifies the link between moms and their children, whether it's by acting out scenes from a favorite book, crafting a movement tale, or taking part in themed exercises based on a narrative.

Holiday- and Seasonally-inspired Activities

Activities that are themed around the seasons and holidays provide interest and diversity to mother-child bonding moments. The guide offers suggestions for seasonal and holiday-appropriate activities that integrate festive themes with physical fitness. Seasonal activities provide a fun and themed way to be active all year long. Examples include snowball battles, pumpkin picking, obstacle courses with holiday themes, and springtime scavenger hunts.

Promoting Optimistic Views on Fitness

Playful activities that combine with physical fitness promote favorable attitudes toward an active lifestyle, which is another benefit of including them into mother-child bonding. The manual places a strong emphasis on the value of early on fostering a pleasant and good association with physical activity. Mothers can give their children a lifelong respect for exercise and well-being by presenting fitness as an enjoyable and shared activity.

Being Adaptable and Flexible in Playful Activities

Understanding that family relationships are dynamic and always changing, the book emphasizes the value of adaptability and flexibility when introducing playful activities. Plans may need to be adjusted in response to life's unforeseen events, and having an open mind encourages flexibility and a positive outlook. Being adaptable guarantees that engaging in playful activities to foster mother-child bonding stays a joyful and stress-free experience.

Creating Enduring Recollections

Finally, "Fit and Fun: Incorporating Playful Activities for Mother-Child Bonding" highlights how play may foster creativity, physical fitness, and a stronger mother-child attachment. Moms can create enduring memories while encouraging their children to lead active and healthy lifestyles by customizing activities based on their child's age and development, going on indoor and outdoor adventures, integrating dance and movement, taking on fitness challenges, incorporating educational elements, embracing water play, practicing yoga and mindfulness, engaging in partner workouts, creating positive attitudes towards fitness, and staying flexible.

The guide understands that the moments of joy and laughter shared via fun activities improve the experience of parenthood. Moms that embrace play not only support their child's physical development but also help them create priceless memories that will last a lifetime. In a vibrant and loving partnership, fitness and enjoyment merge, creating a strong basis for an active and healthy future.

Chapter 8:
Mastering Mom Time: Efficient Workouts for Busy Schedules

Being a mother is a challenging and complex journey that frequently leaves little time for interests outside of work, such as exercising. "Mastering Mom Time: Efficient Workouts for Busy Schedules" discusses the particular difficulties moms encounter in fitting exercise into their schedules while juggling the responsibilities of raising a family. This in-depth manual delves into realistic and time-saving exercise techniques that enable moms to put their health first and fit efficient workouts into their hectic schedules.

Understanding the Time Restrictions

The first thing the guide acknowledges is that mothers frequently have limited time. Long training sessions are difficult to fit in when juggling obligations like childcare, housework, and possibly job. Comprehending the necessity for effective and feasible exercise methods lays the groundwork for developing exercise regimens that suit the demands of a hectic mother's schedule.

Accepting Quick and Vigorous Workouts

When looking for effective fitness within a limited time frame, busy mothers can find great value in short, intense workouts. The notion of high-intensity interval training (HIIT) and other workout forms that save time are introduced in this guide. These exercises are great for mothers who want to get as much exercise as possible within their restricted time; they optimize calorie burn, improve cardiovascular fitness, and build strength in a shorter amount of time.

Tabata Training: A Brief Splash of Vigor

A type of HIIT called tabata training offers an organized and time-saving method of working out. The Tabata protocol—which alternates short bursts of intense activity with rest intervals—is described in the handbook. Because of its versatility, Tabata may be used for a variety of workouts, including strength and aerobic training as well as bodyweight exercises. Moms can get a good exercise in as little as four minutes by including Tabata into their hectic routine.

Effective Bodyweight Exercises

Bodyweight exercises have the benefit of being done in the comfort of one's own home with little need for special equipment. With a variety of effective bodyweight exercises that focus on various muscle groups, the guide offers a full-body workout without the need for complex equipment. These exercises are easy for moms to add into short regimens, providing a comprehensive and time-effective approach to strength training.

Fast Cardio Workouts: Maximizing Every Minute

Cardiovascular exercise is essential for general health, and a busy mom's schedule can easily incorporate short cardio workouts. The guide provides mothers with the ability to select cardiac exercises that suit their fitness levels and preferences by examining both high-impact and low-impact possibilities. Short aerobic bursts, such as jumping jacks, stair climbing, or brisk walks, increase heart rate, speed up metabolism, and help burn calories effectively.

Functional Exercise Programs: Including Exercise in Everyday Activities

Exercise is incorporated into regular jobs using functional workouts, which allow fitness to be smoothly integrated with everyday tasks. The manual offers suggestions for adding exercise to everyday routines like as playing with kids and doing chores around the house. Without the need for dedicated gym sessions, mothers can make the most of their time and include exercise into their daily routine by viewing everyday activities as chances for physical activity.

Fast Exercises for Quiet Times or Naps

The best times to fit in a fast workout for kids are during naps or other quiet times in their routine. The manual looks at ways to make the most of these fleeting times. Moms should prioritize their well-being by making the most of these peaceful moments by working out with focus, adding stretching and flexibility exercises, or performing mindfulness exercises.

A Brief Introduction to Micro-Workouts Throughout the Day Micro-workouts are little spurts of physical activity spaced out throughout the day. In order to make their fitness regimen more manageable and flexible enough to fit into a hectic schedule, the advice advises women to divide it up into smaller sections. A short walk, a fast set of bodyweight exercises, or a few minutes of stretching can all be considered micro-workouts that add up to the required daily physical activity.

Using Online Resources and Workout Apps

Workout applications and internet resources provide busy moms handy answers in the digital era. The benefits of using fitness apps that provide brief, guided workouts are examined in the guide. These apps provide moms with access to efficient workouts at their convenience, ranging from focused bodyweight exercises to quick cardio routines. They also accommodate a variety of fitness levels and preferences.

Building a Home Workout: Affordably and Easily Achievable

Even with a little area, starting a home gym might be a useful tactic for working mothers. The article offers advice on how to set up a basic, reasonably priced home gym with necessary supplies like yoga mats, dumbbells, and resistance bands. A home gym is a useful way to fit exercise into a busy schedule because it removes the need to travel to a fitness center.

Including Strength Training for Effective Outcomes

Increased metabolism, better muscular tone, and increased functional fitness are just a few advantages of strength training. The effectiveness of adding strength training to a busy mom's exercise regimen is emphasized in the guide. Strength training sessions that are brief and concentrated, concentrating on key muscle areas, yield effective outcomes and enhance general physical toughness.

Setting Self-Care First: A Conscious Approach to Exercise

Setting aside time for self-care among the rigors of parenthood is crucial for general wellbeing. The manual advises moms to take a conscious approach to fitness, seeing physical activity as a way to take care of themselves rather than as an extra chore. Mothers can change their perspective and emphasize fitness as a crucial part of their self-care regimen by realizing the psychological and physical advantages of regular exercise.

Making Workout Appointments Non-Negotiable

Making fitness appointments that are non-negotiable is a key component of effective time management. The manual offers methods for setting priorities and time allocation during workout sessions in a hectic schedule. Moms can create a consistent exercise regimen that fits into their daily schedule by giving their workouts the same priority as other commitments.

Accompanying Other Mothers to Ensure Accountability

Maintaining a regular exercise regimen depends heavily on accountability. The manual advises women to collaborate with other mothers in order to build a network of support that inspires dedication and drive. Mothers may increase their accountability and make fitness a fun and team effort by working out together, setting and sharing fitness goals, and supporting one another.

Seeking Expert Advice for Effective Exercise

Seeking expert advice might be helpful for moms looking for individualized and effective exercise regimens. The book looks at the possibility of working with fitness experts, such online coaches or personal trainers, who can create workout regimens specifically suited to the tastes, schedule, and fitness objectives of a busy mother.

Recuperation After Exercise: Increasing Effectiveness

Effective post-workout recovery techniques should be used in conjunction with efficient workouts. The manual offers advice on easy and efficient recuperation techniques, such as stretching, drinking plenty of water, and controlling your diet. Setting recovery as a top priority helps moms maintain their workout regimen without sacrificing their general health.

Including Exercises That Are Family-Friendly

Fitness environments that are inclusive and fun are fostered via family-friendly workouts. The manual offers suggestions on how to include kids in fitness regimens and make working out a family pastime. Moms can help their kids develop a good association with exercise by organizing family dance parties, going on outdoor adventures, or participating in fun fitness challenges.

Precaution vs. Effort: Establishing Durable Routines

When fitting effective workouts into a busy schedule, consistency is essential. The manual places a strong emphasis on creating enduring habits by recommending regular exercise over intense but infrequent sessions. Mothers who regularly work out efficiently might get cumulative benefits that support their long-term health and wellbeing.

Honoring Little Victories: Inspiration for the Path

Maintaining motivation during the fitness journey requires acknowledging and celebrating minor victories. The manual urges moms to celebrate their accomplishments, whether it's doing a fast workout on a hectic day or regularly adhering to a fitness regimen. Honoring these successes promotes optimism and emphasizes how crucial it is to put self-care first.

In conclusion, enabling mothers to manage their time well Finally,

"Mastering Mom Time: Efficient Workouts for Busy Schedules" is a useful manual for moms who want to put their health first yet have a busy schedule.

Time management strategies such as acknowledging time constraints, embracing quick and intense workouts, incorporating Tabata training, engaging in effective bodyweight exercises, making every minute count with quick cardio sessions, incorporating exercise into daily activities, using quiet times and naps for workouts, introducing micro-workouts throughout the day, utilizing online workout resources and workout apps, setting up a home gym, incorporating strength training, putting self-care first, making workouts non-negotiable appointments, collaborating with other mothers for accountability, seeking expert advice, emphasizing post-workout recovery, incorporating family-friendly workouts, and celebrating little victories, mothers have the ability to take control of their time and accept effective exercise as a long-term and essential component of their hectic lifestyles.

The author acknowledges that motherhood is a dynamic journey and that finding time for exercise calls for flexibility and inventiveness. Mothers can prioritize their health, increase their energy, and provide a positive example for their families by using effective exercise routines. Gaining control over mom time is the first step toward improved health, increased physical toughness, and a balanced, purposeful existence.

Chapter 9:
Overcoming Obstacles: Resilience in the Face of Challenges

Life is a convoluted journey with many of twists and turns, and challenges can occasionally show up as formidable obstacles. The book "Overcoming Obstacles: Resilience in the Face of Challenges" explores both the intrinsic resilience of humans and the transformative power of overcoming adversity. This comprehensive study examines the characteristics of obstacles, the psychological foundations of resilience, and practical methods for fostering and strengthening resilience in the face of hardship.

Knowing the Different Types of Barriers

Obstacles abound in the human experience and can take many different forms, such as social problems, unanticipated tragedies, and personal setbacks. The manual begins by urging readers to be aware of the range of obstacles they may face and emphasizing that they are opportunities for growth and development rather than insurmountable obstacles. By acknowledging that obstacles do exist, people may shift their perspective from viewing challenges as roadblocks to resilience to viewing them as stepping stones.

The Resilience Psychology

Resilience is a psychological and emotional quality that allows people to learn from their experiences, adjust to change, and overcome adversity. The handbook delves into the psychological underpinnings of resilience, covering concepts like growth mindset, optimism, and self-efficacy. Knowing these components enables people to see resilience as a skill rather than a fixed attribute that can be cultivated and nurtured.

Adopting a Growth Perspective

A growth mindset, which promotes the idea that setbacks present chances for growth and learning, is a fundamental component of resilience. The manual presents the idea of a growth mentality, stressing the significance of developing an attitude that sees obstacles as opportunities for improvement and failures as transitory. People can change their story from one of helplessness to one of empowerment by adopting a growth mindset, which builds resilience in the face of adversity.

The Part Optimism Plays in Resilience

Resilience is greatly influenced by optimism, which molds people's perspectives and reactions to adversity. The handbook examines the value of keeping a cheerful attitude in the face of hardship. Those who are optimistic typically view setbacks as momentary and situational, which enable them to face challenges with confidence in their capacity to overcome barriers. Reframing negative thoughts and emphasizing strengths are two tactics for cultivating optimism that help build resilience.

Developing Self-Efficacy: Positivity about One's Capabilities

One of the main elements of resilience is self-efficacy, or the conviction that one can control events and consequences. The handbook highlights the importance of self-efficacy in overcoming obstacles and exhorts readers to grow in self-awareness and self-assurance. Developing self-efficacy entails recognizing one's own accomplishments, setting achievable goals, and dividing work into manageable steps. Increasing self-efficacy helps people develop a resilient mindset, which empowers them to take on obstacles head-on and confidently.

The Development of Emotional Intelligence
Resilience is closely linked to emotional intelligence, which is the capacity to identify, comprehend, and control one's emotions. The relationship between emotional intelligence and the ability to overcome challenges is examined by the guide. The process of increasing self-awareness, self-regulation, empathy, and successful interpersonal skills is known as emotional intelligence cultivation. Through comprehending and managing emotions when confronted with difficulties, people can improve their resilience and sustain a well-rounded and flexible reaction to misfortune.

Gratitude and Flexibility
The capacity to adjust to shifting conditions and acknowledge the truth of a situation is a key component of resilience. The manual places a strong emphasis on the value of acceptance and flexibility in overcoming challenges. Acceptance does not mean giving up; rather, it is seeing the situation as it is and enabling people to focus their energies on positive solutions. Being adaptable entails having an open mind, changing course as necessary, and coming up with substitute ideas. People build resilience that helps them deal with life's unpredictability by accepting acceptance and flexibility.

Gaining Knowledge from Misfortune: Recovery from Trauma
When faced with adversity with fortitude, progress can occur after the trauma. In introducing the idea of post-traumatic growth, the guide emphasizes the transformational process that takes place when people face and overcome obstacles. People can come out of adversity stronger, more empathetic, and with a greater sense of purpose rather than being defined by it alone.

Resilience that goes beyond survival is developed and personal growth is sparked by learning from hardship.

Building Up Social Support Systems

One of the most effective tools for creating and maintaining resilience is social support. The handbook examines how social networks might support people in overcoming obstacles. Robust social support systems offer a feeling of community, practical help, and emotional support. Building strong bonds with friends, family, and the community promotes resilience by acting as a safety net in trying circumstances. People who have strong social ties are better able to overcome challenges with the help of others.

Reduced Stress and Mindfulness

Building resilience can be facilitated by practicing mindfulness, which is the art of being totally present and involved in the present moment. The manual presents mindfulness as a way to lessen stress, develop self-awareness, and strengthen emotional control. Deep breathing exercises and other mindfulness techniques enable people to respond to difficulties with more calm and clarity. People can increase their resilience by practicing mindfulness, which increases their awareness of their thoughts and feelings.

Establishing Reasonable Objectives and Making Gradual Progress

Creating attainable objectives and breaking them down into doable chunks is a useful tactic for developing resilience. Setting realistic goals is crucial, according to the advice, both for personal and professional endeavors. Larger problems can be divided into smaller, more doable activities so that people still feel in control and accomplished. Honoring small victories strengthens the idea that conquering challenges is a methodical and steady process and promotes a positive outlook.

Seeking Expert Assistance When Required

In some circumstances, getting expert assistance is a proactive step toward developing resilience. The handbook urges people to identify situations in which seeking outside help—such as counseling or therapy—may be advantageous. Professional support offers a secure environment where people can explore their feelings, create coping mechanisms, and learn how to overcome certain obstacles. Asking for assistance when required is a show of strength and a useful tool in the process of developing resilience.

Preserving Physical Well-Being Emotional and mental resilience are strongly associated with physical well-being. The handbook emphasizes the value of upholding a healthy lifestyle, which includes consistent exercise, a balanced diet, and enough sleep. Physical health increases energy, lowers stress, and lifts the spirits, all of which support overall resilience. Making physical health self-care a priority builds resilience, which enables people to deal with life's obstacles more effectively.

Adopting an Adaptable Mentality

A flexible attitude is able to respond to changing circumstances, see opportunities in setbacks, and modify objectives as necessary. The manual delves into the idea of adopting a flexible attitude, stressing the importance of changing with the times. People that possess a flexible mindset approach issues with an open mind and are willing to consider alternative options, as opposed to strictly following preconceived conceptions or plans. This adaptive strategy builds a willingness to consider other options when presented with challenges, which enhances resilience.

Thinking Back on One's Past Resilience and Personal Strengths

It can be inspiring and motivating to think back on prior examples of perseverance and personal qualities. The manual helps people identify their innate abilities and think back to instances when they overcame difficulties. Recognizing past resiliency helps people feel more confident about their capacity to get past present challenges. Thinking back on one's own strengths helps one remember that resilience is a dynamic, ever-evolving trait that belongs to each individual.

In summary, strengthening the human spirit

To sum up, "Overcoming Obstacles: Resilience in the Face of Challenges" offers guidance to those who want to develop and fortify their resilience along the complex journey that is life. People may empower themselves to face challenges with courage and tenacity by comprehending the nature of obstacles, adopting a growth mindset, encouraging optimism, developing self-efficacy, cultivating emotional intelligence, accepting and adapting to change, learning from adversity, nurturing social support networks, practicing mindfulness, setting realistic goals, seeking professional support when necessary, maintaining physical well-being, adopting a flexible mindset, thinking back on personal strengths, and realizing the transformative potential of resilience.

The handbook acknowledges that resilience is the capacity to overcome and negotiate adversity rather than the absence of it. Every challenge is a chance for personal development, and through building resilience, people can turn adversity into a driving force for growth. "Overcoming Obstacles" turns into a monument to the human spirit's unwavering perseverance, which enables people to overcome adversity and come out stronger, smarter, and more resilient than before.

Chapter 10:
Holistic Wellness: Mind-Body Practices for Resilient Motherhood

First of all,

Being a mother is a life-changing experience that involves happiness, difficulties, and a range of feelings. Mothers' health has to be nurtured in a comprehensive way that incorporates the mind and body. The book "Holistic Wellness: Mind-Body Practices for Resilient Motherhood" delves into the ways in which mind-body techniques might improve mothers' resilience. This thorough manual explores the relationship between mental and physical health, offering helpful tips and techniques to promote overall wellness during the transition to motherhood.

Comprehending Holistic Health:

In order to attain a condition of harmony and balance, holistic wellness includes the combination of mental, emotional, and physical well-being. The tutorial starts out by highlighting how the mind and body are intertwined, highlighting the idea that taking care of one affects the other. A robust and successful mothering experience necessitates attending to both the physical and emotional aspects of well-being, as holistic wellness acknowledges.

Mind-Body Connection:

A key component of holistic wellbeing is the mind-body connection. The guide highlights how thoughts and emotions can affect how the body functions as it examines the complex interplay between mental and physical health. Understanding the relationship between the mind and body enables moms to implement techniques that enhance balance between the two, so improving general wellbeing.

Mindfulness Techniques for now-Moment Living:
By bringing mothers into the now, mindfulness techniques promote acceptance and awareness. The manual presents attentive parenting methods, deep breathing exercises, and mindfulness meditation. Mothers can develop resilience by managing stress, improving focus, and appreciating the richness of every moment in their motherhood experience by implementing mindfulness into their daily lives.

Yoga for Mental and Physical Balance:
Yoga integrates meditation, breath work, and physical postures into a complete practice. In examining the advantages of yoga for moms, the guide emphasizes the practice's capacity to improve mental clarity, strength, and flexibility. Adding yoga to a mother's schedule creates a space for self-care, rest, and renewal, which benefits her physical and emotional health.

Body Awareness and Self-Compassion:
Two of the most important aspects of holistic wellness are body awareness and self-compassion. Recognizing the changes and difficulties that come with childbirth, the guide encourages moms to develop a good relationship with their bodies. By treating oneself with kindness and understanding, self-compassion practice cultivates a resilient and nurturing mindset.

Relaxation techniques for managing stress:
The responsibilities of parenting can lead to stress, which can have negative effects on one's physical and emotional well-being. The manual presents many methods of relaxation, including guided imagery, progressive muscle

relaxation, and aromatherapy. These techniques provide moms the tools they need to properly manage their stress, encouraging composure and fortitude in the face of everyday obstacles.

Emotional Resilience and Positive Psychology:
The capacity to adjust and overcome hardship is known as emotional resilience. The manual examines positive psychology concepts, placing special emphasis on cultivating positive emotions, optimism, and thankfulness. Mothers can improve their emotional resilience and cultivate a positive outlook that enhances general well-being by adopting positive psychology techniques into their daily life.

Nutritional Sourcing for vigor and Energy:
Food is essential for maintaining good physical and mental health. The manual offers advice on how to fuel the body with a diet that is both well-balanced and nutrient-rich. Whole foods, water, and mindful eating are nutritional habits that support resilient parenting by promoting long-term energy, mental clarity, and general vigor.

Sleep hygiene and restoration:
Getting enough sleep is essential for maintaining good physical and mental health. The handbook places a strong emphasis on moms' need for restful sleep and good sleep hygiene. Helpful advice on setting up habits for nighttime and building a sleep-friendly atmosphere can increase the quality of sleep, boost resilience, and advance general wellness.

Connection and Community Support:
In addition to individual practices, holistic wellness also includes relationships and community support. The handbook emphasizes how important it is to look for social relationships and create a support system. Creating a feeling of community through interactions with other like-

minded mothers, experience sharing, and mutual support helps mothers become more emotionally resilient.

Bonding and Mindful Parenting:

Mindful parenting entails being totally present and involved in the parenting process. The handbook looks at techniques including purposeful bonding activities, nonjudgmental awareness, and active listening that promote a mindful parenting style. The mother-child bond is strengthened by mindful parenting, which supports a strong and supportive family unit.

Effective time management and prioritization are essential to a mother's overall well-being in parenting. The manual offers doable methods for allocating tasks, establishing limits, and designing a well-rounded plan. Mothers who are good at managing their time can minimize stress, maximize output, and make time for self-care activities that improve their general wellbeing.

Using Creativity and Expression to Release Emotions:

Self-discovery and emotional release can be achieved via creative expression. The manual urges moms to experiment with artistic endeavors like painting, music, or journaling as a way to communicate their feelings and build resilience. Creative endeavors offer a healing environment for introspection and emotional digestion.

Outdoor Activities and Nature Connection:

Taking part in outdoor activities and establishing a connection with nature are beneficial to one's physical and mental health. The benefits of being outside, whether on walks, hikes, or playing outside with kids, are discussed in the guide. Connecting with nature fosters calm, reduces stress, and increases one's sense of interconnection with the surroundings.

Therapy and expert Support:

Taking the initiative to pursue holistic wellness means seeking out expert assistance. The handbook emphasizes how crucial it is to get in touch with therapists or mental health specialists when necessary. Mothers who seek professional support can explore their feelings and ideas in a private setting, learn coping mechanisms, and receive guidance in overcoming obstacles.

Frequent Medical Examinations and Preventive Care:

Proactive health management is essential to holistic wellbeing. The need of routine health examinations and preventive care is emphasized in the guide. Resilience in motherhood is facilitated by keeping an eye on physical health, swiftly resolving issues, and placing a high priority on preventive measures. All of these behaviors contribute to overall well-being.

Creating Healthy limits for Self-Care:

An essential part of holistic wellbeing is creating healthy limits. The handbook exhorts moms to set firm limits that put their own health and well-being first. Establishing boundaries entails establishing space for relaxation and renewal, articulating requirements clearly, and saying no when it's essential.

In summary:

To sum up,

"Holistic Wellness: Mind-Body Practices for Resilient Motherhood" is an all-inclusive manual for moms who want to take a holistic approach to nurturing their well-being.

Mothers can experience resilient and flourishing motherhood by acknowledging the interconnectedness of mental and physical health, incorporating mindfulness practices, embracing yoga, fostering body awareness, effectively managing stress, cultivating emotional resilience, prioritizing nutritional nourishment, focusing on sleep hygiene, forming connections, engaging in mindful parenting, managing time efficiently, pursuing creative outlets, connecting with nature, seeking professional support, and setting boundaries for self-care.

Mothers who practice holistic wellbeing are more equipped to handle the challenges of their roles with grace, resiliency, and a keen sense of self. Mothers can create resilience, balance, and general well-being by adopting mind-body activities. These advantages extend beyond the mothers themselves, as they can also have a significant impact on the well-being of their families. Mothers find a transforming approach in the field of holistic wellness that recognizes the nuances of their journey and promotes a resilient and powerful state of being.

Chapter 11:
Partnering for Fitness: Engaging the Family in a Healthy Lifestyle

First of all,

It can be difficult to find time for exercise and a healthy lifestyle in the fast-paced modern world, particularly for families balancing multiple commitments. The book "Partnering for Fitness: Engaging the Family in a Healthy Lifestyle" delves at the life-changing potential of enlisting the whole family in the quest for health. This in-depth manual explores the value of teamwork, the advantages of shared activities, and doable tactics to establish a nurturing atmosphere that encourages physical health and a well-rounded lifestyle for the whole family.

Acknowledging the Importance of Family Fitness:

Family fitness promotes a shared commitment to health, fortifies bonds, and establishes a supporting framework for all parties involved. It goes beyond individual well-being. The handbook highlights the importance of making exercise a group effort and acknowledges the critical role families play in shaping habits, encouraging a positive outlook, and imparting values connected to health and well-being that last a lifetime.

Creating a Supportive atmosphere:

The cornerstone of family fitness is the establishment of a supportive atmosphere. The handbook looks at ways to create an environment that promotes physical activity and healthy decisions. Setting the foundation for family fitness requires deliberate efforts to build a healthy home environment that emphasizes wholesome food choices and active living, as well as open conversation about health objectives.

Establishing Family-Based Health Objectives:
Establishing family-based health objectives fosters a feeling of common direction and drive. Families are encouraged by the book to jointly determine fitness and health goals while taking into account the individual needs and preferences of each family member. Families can reinforce the idea that well-being is a team effort by creating a roadmap for their fitness journey through the establishment of specific and attainable goals.

Family-Friendly Physical Activities: Taking part in family-friendly physical activities makes working out fun and something you all do together. The guide offers a range of activities that are appropriate for people of all ages, including sports, hiking, biking, family outings, and swimming. In addition to improving physical health, these activities foster teamwork, make enduring memories, and deepen the bonds within the family.

Fitting Exercise Into Daily Routines: Including exercise in daily routines is a doable way to promote family heath. The book looks at how to incorporate exercise into daily living in a natural way. Some ideas include using the stairs, choosing active transportation, or working out for brief periods of time with a partner. Families may overcome time constraints and prioritize health in the midst of busy schedules by incorporating activity into everyday routines.

Family Fitness Challenges:
Including family fitness challenges in health goals brings a lighthearted and pleasant competitive element. The manual advises designing tasks that accommodate the family's wide range of interests and fitness levels. Family fitness challenges, whether they involve a weekly fitness goal, a step challenge, or a friendly sports competition, encourage involvement, increase motivation, and create a sense of accomplishment.

Meal Planning and Healthy Cooking Together:
Including the family in meal planning and cooking raises nutritional knowledge. Nutrition is an essential part of living a healthy lifestyle. The cookbook delves into the advantages of cooking with one another, inspiring families to try out new recipes, sample different cuisines, and decide on wholesome meals as a group. Families teach their children important culinary skills and foster an appreciation for healthful, home-cooked meals by getting them involved in the kitchen.

Mindful Eating Techniques:
Mindful eating encourages a balanced relationship with food and increases awareness of food choices. The handbook presents mindful eating techniques, urging families to enjoy meals together, tune out outside distractions, and pay attention to their bodies' signals of hunger and fullness. Families that practice mindful eating boost not just physical wellness but also enhance the overall dining experience.

Family Outdoor Adventures:
Spending time outdoors with nature is a fun and exciting way for families to keep active. The book advises becoming involved in outdoor pursuits like hiking, camping, picnics, and nature hikes. In addition to improving physical health, these excursions provide a chance for family time, exploration, and a respite from the stresses of everyday life.

Using Technology to Improve Family Fitness:
Using technology to improve family fitness can make it more accessible and interesting. The use of wearable technology, interactive video games, and fitness applications to encourage physical activity is covered in the guide. Through thoughtful integration of technology, families can transform screen time into active time,

promoting equilibrium between digital interaction and physical health.

Creating a Family Exercise Program:

Having a regular family workout program gives your kids structure and reinforces good behavior. Making a weekly schedule with specific hours for exercise, meal prep, and relaxation is advised by the guide. Establishing family exercise as a routine helps to solidify the commitment to a healthy lifestyle by integrating it into everyday life.

Honoring Milestones and Achievements:

Highlighting the good aspects of the fitness journey is done best when done as a family. Families are encouraged by the book to recognize and celebrate both individual and group achievements. Recognizing accomplishments makes the family feel proud and motivated, whether it's completing a fitness goal, attempting a new activity, or changing their food habits.

Opportunities for Health Literacy Education:

Increasing health literacy within the family improves knowledge and consciousness of wellness concepts. The handbook places a strong emphasis on teaching family members the advantages of consistent exercise, a healthy diet, and general wellbeing. Fostering health literacy helps families make educated decisions, create a common language about health, and provide each member the tools they need to actively participate in their own well-being.

Making Sleep a Family Priority:

Getting enough sleep is essential for good health, and making sleep a priority requires cooperation from the whole family. The handbook covers methods for establishing regular sleep schedules, making a sleep environment that is family-friendly, and emphasizing the value of getting enough good sleep for everyone. Families may support good physical and emotional well-being by making sleep a priority.

Getting Professional Advice: In some circumstances, getting professional advice can improve family fitness programs. Families are encouraged by the recommendations to seek advice from medical professionals, dietitians, or fitness specialists as needed. Expert counsel is customized, deals with particular health issues, and guarantees that family exercise programs complement personal objectives.

Cultivating a Positive Family Attitude:

Maintaining a healthy lifestyle requires cultivating a positive family attitude. The book delves into the efficacy of encouraging words, mutual goals, and a loving disposition among family members. Families that foster a positive outlook foster an atmosphere that supports resilience, encourages individual growth, and reaffirms the idea that leading a healthy lifestyle can be both pleasant and attainable.

Family Reflection and review:

Families are better able to evaluate and make the required changes to their fitness journey when they engage in regular reflection and review. Families are encouraged by the guide to have candid conversations about their experiences, difficulties, and accomplishments. Through collaborative reflection, families can improve their methods, establish fresh objectives, and continually modify their fitness regimens to suit the changing requirements of every family member.

In summary,

 "Partnering for Fitness: Engaging the Family in a Healthy Lifestyle"

offers families a road map for starting a journey towards well-being as a group. Families can develop a sustainable and all-encompassing approach to health by appreciating the value of family fitness, creating a supportive environment, defining group health goals, planning and preparing healthy meals together, taking part in challenges, incorporating technology mindfully, planning and cooking healthy meals, practicing mindful eating, enjoying outdoor adventures, promoting health literacy, prioritizing sleep, developing a positive family mindset, and reflecting on a regular basis.

Family fitness involves more than simply physical activity; it also involves building relationships, establishing healthy routines, and establishing an atmosphere that is encouraging and beneficial to all family members. Families may handle the difficulties of contemporary living while laying the groundwork for a stronger, healthier, and more resilient future by working together and committing to well-being. Joining forces for fitness turns a relationship into a shared journey that improves people's lives on the inside as well as the outside, encouraging a lifetime dedication to health and wellbeing.

Chapter 12:
Ages and Stages: Adapting Fitness Routines to Motherhood Transitions

Being a mother is a dynamic journey filled with many changes, each of which has its own pleasures and challenges. The thorough manual "Ages and Stages: Adapting Fitness Routines to Motherhood Transitions" delves into the significance of modifying exercise regimens to correspond with the changing phases of motherhood. Throughout the many phases of motherhood, this guide offers moms useful ideas and techniques to support them in embracing a flexible and sustainable approach to fitness. Topics covered include pregnancy, postpartum recovery, and the difficulties of raising multiple age groups.

Embracing Pregnancy exercise:
Being pregnant is a life-changing experience that calls for a customized approach to exercise. In order to help pregnant moms' physical and mental wellbeing, the guide highlights the significance of embracing pregnancy fitness. Low-impact workouts, including swimming and yoga for pregnant women, can preserve strength and flexibility while reducing joint stress. Exercises for the pelvic floor and mild strength training can help to improve general fitness and get the body ready for childbirth.

Postpartum Recovery and Gradual Reentry:
Gradual reentry into fitness is necessary after postpartum recovery, which is a crucial stage. The manual emphasizes how crucial it is to pay attention to your body's signals and ease back into physical activity after giving birth. Rebuilding core strength, pelvic floor health, and general

stability are the main goals of postpartum exercise. Walking, light strength training, and postpartum yoga are examples of activities that promote healing and enhance the mother's physical and emotional health.

Managing the Toddler Years:

When their kids get older and more independent, moms must adjust their exercise regimens to meet their changing needs. The manual looks at fun ways to get kids moving, such engaging in interactive play and going outside. Jogging or walking with a stroller offers a chance to get cardiovascular activity and spend time with the child. Moms may embrace their toddlers' energy and achieve their fitness goals by combining planned exercises with unstructured playtime.

Fitness with School-Age Children:

A mother's time is demanded differently during the school-age phase, necessitating flexibility and thoughtful planning. The advice recommends mixing in family-friendly pursuits including organized sports, bicycling, and hiking. Encouraging kids to engage in physical activities promotes a healthy lifestyle that benefits the whole family. Additionally, moms should prioritize their fitness within the limits of hectic schedules by looking for possibilities for quick and effective at-home workouts.

Adolescence and Collaborative Fitness:

Adolescence offers a chance for collaborative fitness, promoting a feeling of bonding between mothers and their developing offspring. The book covers a variety of teen-focused activities, including team sports, fitness classes, and group exercise. Together, working out encourages a healthy lifestyle and offers a platform for candid conversation and closeness during this pivotal adolescent period.

Managing Fitness with Multiple Children:
Managing fitness with multiple children of different ages calls for a planned and inclusive strategy from moms. The book makes recommendations for family-friendly events that suit a range of age ranges so that everyone may take part. With circuit training or interval exercise, moms can effectively manage their time while meeting the many requirements of their children. Mothers can help their children develop lasting habits by modeling a healthy attitude toward fitness as a family value.

Empty Nest exercise and Self-Rediscovery:
When children grow out of the nest, mothers go through a period of self-reflection and exercise turns into a tool for wellbeing and personal development. The manual exhorts moms to establish personal objectives, participate in fitness communities, and try new things. During the empty nest phase, engaging in activities such as hiking alone, taking group lessons, or learning a new sport can enhance physical fitness and promote a sense of fulfillment and self-discovery.

Menopause and Emphasizing Holistic Wellness:
A woman's body experiences hormonal changes during menopause, which necessitates modifications to her exercise regimen. The manual places a strong emphasis on the value of putting holistic wellness—which includes cardiovascular, strength, and flexibility training—first. During this period of transition, practicing mindfulness and yoga can help manage stress and support emotional well-being. Mothers can manage menopause with resilience and vigor if they prioritize self-care and modify their exercise regimens to suit their changing demands.

Changing Exercise Routines to Aging Gracefully:

Changing exercise routines is essential to aging gracefully, which is a normal aspect of life. The manual covers low-impact activities that protect cardiovascular health and are easy on joints, like cycling or swimming. Exercises for flexibility and balance become crucial to avoiding injuries and improving general mobility. Strength training is still essential for maintaining bone density and muscle mass, which helps women, enjoy their golden years with a robust and resilient body.

The Value of Routine Medical Examinations:
Routine checkups with the doctor become essential to overall wellbeing as a mother progresses through the stages of parenting. The need of proactive health management—which includes regular screenings and discussions with medical professionals—is emphasized throughout the guide. Mothers can modify their exercise regimens to better suit their changing health requirements when they undergo routine check-ups, which assist detect any health issues early on.

Personalization and Flexibility in Fitness:
It takes both to tailor exercise regimens to the ups and downs of parenthood. The manual emphasizes how important it is to pay attention to one's body, acknowledge personal preferences, and modify exercises as necessary. Personalization enables moms to customize their fitness journeys to meet their particular situation, guaranteeing that the chosen activities provide happiness, satisfaction, and long-term health advantages.

Managing Motherhood Responsibilities and Self-Care:
Throughout parenthood transitions, striking a balance between self-care and motherhood responsibilities is a crucial subject. The manual covers time management techniques, boundary-setting techniques, and needs communication techniques. Mothers lay a solid basis for

prioritizing their well-being throughout the many phases of motherhood by striking a good balance between their obligations to their families and their own needs.

Creating a Supportive Community:

Navigating the joys and challenges of transitioning into parenthood depends on creating a supportive community. The manual exhorts mothers to make connections with like-minded people via social media, online forums, or neighborhood exercise clubs. moms who are part of a supportive group benefit from encouragement, a sense of camaraderie, and shared experiences that assist them throughout their varied journeys as moms.

Positive affirmations and mindset adjustments:

Adapting exercise regimens to the demands of parenthood requires a strong mentality. The book delves into the effectiveness of mindset changes and positive affirmations in building a resilient and adaptable approach to exercise. Mothers who adopt a positive outlook on life are better equipped to accept change, see obstacles as chances for personal development, and recognize their accomplishments at every phase of parenting.

In conclusion, a lifetime path towards adaptive fitness:

In conclusion, mothers starting a lifetime journey of adaptive fitness might refer to "Ages and Stages: Adapting Fitness Routines to Motherhood Transitions" as a reference. Every stage of motherhood presents its own chances and difficulties, necessitating adaptability, individuality, and a dedication to one's own well-being. Mothers can navigate the many stages of motherhood with resilience, vitality, and a commitment to lifelong health by embracing pregnancy fitness, managing postpartum recovery, incorporating toddlers and school-age children into workouts, participating in collaborative fitness with teenagers, juggling fitness with multiple children, adapting to the empty nest phase, prioritizing holistic wellness during menopause, aging gracefully, attending regular health check-ups, personalizing fitness routines, balancing self-care, creating a supportive community, and encouraging positive mindset shifts.

Transitions to motherhood are dynamic; they are always evolving. Through customization of exercise regimens to meet the various ages and phases of parenting, women can develop a strong and confident bond with their bodies. A mother's quest toward adaptive fitness transforms into a celebration of her strength, an example of her resiliency, and a lifetime dedication to wellbeing that affects her mental, emotional, and spiritual well-being in addition to her physical health.

Chapter 13:
Strong and Sexy: Rediscovering Confidence in Motherhood

Being a mother is a wonderful adventure filled with love, development, and change. Nonetheless, a woman's sense of confidence and self-worth may occasionally be questioned due to the accompanying mental and physical changes. The thorough manual "Strong and Sexy: Rediscovering Confidence in Motherhood" explores the complex facets of confidence, accepting one's body, and developing a good self-image throughout the course of motherhood. The goal of this book is to give moms the confidence and self-assurance they need to face parenting head-on, embrace their strength, and rediscover their sensuality.

Accepting the Changing Body:

Being a mother brings about bodily changes, which are an inevitable aspect of the experience. Mothers are urged by the guidance to accept and love themselves while they adjust to these changes. A positive outlook is fostered by understanding and appreciating the body's capacity to nurture and generate life, from pregnancy to postpartum recuperation. Accepting one's changing body turns into a celebration of fortitude, resiliency, and the wonders of motherhood.

Fitness for Self-Belief and Overall Health:

Fitting exercise into daily life improves not just physical health but also self-esteem and general wellbeing. The benefits of consistent exercise for mood, energy, and body image are discussed in the guide. Dancing, yoga, and strength training are examples of joyful hobbies that promote empowerment and confidence. Being fit turns into a way to express oneself and take back control of one's body and wellbeing.

Fostering Self-Care Habits:

Self-care is essential to having confidence as a mother. The handbook places a strong emphasis on setting aside time for self-care routines that support the body, mind, and soul. Taking care of oneself, whether it is by taking a soothing bath, engaging in mindfulness exercises, or setting aside time for personal interests, enhances one's sense of fulfillment and positive self-perception. Taking care of oneself enables moms to rejuvenate and tackle their responsibilities with revitalized assurance.

Clothes for Confidence:

A woman's self-perception and level of confidence can be greatly influenced by the way she looks. The book delves into the idea of wearing with confidence, advising moms to dress in clothes that give them a sense of ease and empowerment. Developing a positive self-image is facilitated by discovering styles that value uniqueness and improve self-expression. Mothers can express themselves through their clothes, showcasing their individual beauty and sense of style.

Honoring Milestones and Accomplishments:

Being a mother is full of major and minor accomplishments. The manual advises moms to cherish these occasions in order to bolster their sense of self-worth and confidence. Every accomplishment, from a child's first steps to their level of physical condition, is proof of their fortitude and resiliency. Honoring these successes promotes optimism and strengthens the idea that motherhood is a lifelong process of success and development.

Regaining Intimacy and Sensuality:

Regaining intimacy and sensuality is essential to feeling confident as a mother. The manual recognizes the significance of preserving a relationship with one's intimacy and sensuality in the face of evolving physical and lifestyle changes. Finding new methods to express sensuality, prioritizing personal times, and keeping lines of communication open with your spouse all help you maintain a positive self-image and a happy love relationship. In the context of parenting, rediscovering pleasure turns into a voyage of self-discovery and connection.

Developing a Positive Self-Image:

Developing a positive self-image is developing an attitude that regards and honors oneself. The manual covers techniques for changing negative self-talk to positive ones, emphasizing strengths, and engaging in self-compassion exercises. Developing a healthy self-image is a continuous process that requires accepting the many facets that make each mother special and precious as well as realizing one's value beyond outward appearances.

Seeking Support and Connection:

Having a strong support system and feeling connected to others can help boost confidence. The manual advises moms to look for assistance from friends, relatives, or support groups so they can exchange stories, struggles, and victories. Making connections with people who are familiar with the experience of parenting offers comfort and a sense of unity. Seeking assistance turns into a useful tool for establishing and preserving confidence.

Mindfulness and Body Positivity:

Developing self-confidence can be greatly enhanced by engaging in mindfulness practices and adopting body positivity. The manual explains mindfulness concepts and exhorts moms to accept their bodies as they are and live in the present. Rejecting irrational social norms and appreciating the variety of body types are key components of embracing body positivity. Mothers can overcome the difficulties associated with body image with confidence and self-love by cultivating a thoughtful and body-positive mindset.

Expert Advice for Self-Transformation:
Depending on the circumstances, getting expert advice can help with confidence-boosting and self-transformation. The handbook recognizes the need of life coaches, therapists, and fitness experts who focus on women's health. Expert advice provides specialized techniques for conquering certain obstacles, encouraging self-discovery, and confidently negotiating the intricacies of parenthood.

Time management and Prioritization:
When obligations and personal interests are balanced, confidence frequently blossoms. The manual looks at time management and prioritization techniques that work. Establishing boundaries, planning routines that accommodate self-care, and appreciating the value of alone time are all components of a confident and well-rounded approach to motherhood. Effective time management becomes essential to preserving a positive self-image while carrying out multiple responsibilities.

Positive Role Modeling for Children:
Motherhood is about more than just one's own wellbeing; it's about setting an example for the future generation. The handbook places a strong emphasis on the value of providing kids with positive role models who exhibit body positivity, self-love, and confidence. Mothers who exhibit these traits enable their kids to develop resilience, confidence, and positive body and self-worth relationships.

Accepting Change and Resilience:

Being a mother is a journey marked by constant change, which calls for resilience and flexibility. The handbook delves into the idea of accepting change and seeing it as a chance for personal development. Developing adaptation builds resilience and elegance in negotiating the changing dynamics of parenthood. As mothers negotiate the difficulties and rewards of every new situation, accepting change becomes a pillar of confidence.

Honoring Individuality:

Every mother is different, possessing her own qualities, charms, and strengths. The handbook highlights the value of appreciating uniqueness as a basis for self-assurance. Positivity regarding one's physical and personal attributes is enhanced by acknowledging and appreciating them. Honoring individuality enables moms to approach motherhood genuinely and with confidence.

Including Playfulness and Fun:

 Despite the obligations of motherhood, it's important to keep a positive, upbeat attitude by including playfulness and fun. The handbook recommends doing joyful things, including dancing, playing with kids, or pursuing artistic endeavors. Having fun and being playful promotes positivity and builds resilience and confidence in the face of day-to-day obstacles.

Self-Reflection and Personal Development:

Developing confidence as a mother entails a process of introspection and development. Mothers are encouraged by the guide to take stock of their journey, recognize their own successes, and pinpoint areas in which they still need to grow. Accepting personal development is a sign of fortitude and resiliency, and it helps foster a changing self-awareness that fits the changing demands of parenthood.

Final Thoughts: A Path of Self-Love and Empowerment

Finally,

"Strong and Sexy: Rediscovering Confidence in Motherhood" is a manual for moms who want to go on a path of self-love and empowerment.

Being confident is a dynamic quality that develops with self-acceptance and self-discovery rather than a static trait. Mothers can successfully navigate the challenges of motherhood with confidence, resilience, and a strong sense of self-love if they embrace the evolving body, incorporate fitness for well-being, nurture self-care practices, dress for confidence, celebrate milestones, rediscover sensuality, build a positive self-image, seek support, practice mindfulness, embrace body positivity, seek professional guidance, manage time effectively, set positive examples for their children, embrace change, celebrate individuality, incorporate fun, and encourage introspection and personal growth.

Regaining confidence is a significant and continuous process that goes hand in hand with how motherhood transforms. Mothers who embrace femininity, strength, and self-determination improve their own wellbeing and leave a healthy legacy for the next generation. "Strong and Sexy" turns into a proclamation of empowerment and self-love, encouraging moms to celebrate their strength, accept their individual beauty, and face parenthood with courage, fortitude, and a dazzling sense of self.

Conclusion:
The Ever-Resilient Mother - A Lifetime of Physical Strength

The wide range of duties and obligations that women take on throughout motherhood make it an incredibly meaningful experience. In the face of both happiness and difficulties, moms frequently exhibit incredible fortitude and bravery. The documentary "The Ever-Resilient Mother - A Lifetime of Physical Strength" explores the physical resilience that mothers demonstrate at different points in their lives. From the initial stages of gestation to the golden years of old age, this manual honors the continuous physical fortitude journey that characterizes the essence of motherhood.

Pregnancy and the Foundations of Strength:
The amazing process of being pregnant marks the start of the road to physical strength. The transforming quality of a woman's body during this time is emphasized by the guide. Pregnancy creates the groundwork for moms' enduring resilience, from the early phases of supporting a developing life to the resilience of labor and delivery. Prenatal exercise, such as weight training and mild yoga, not only promotes a healthy pregnancy but also lays the physical groundwork for the challenges that lie ahead.

Postpartum Recuperation and the Emergence of Strength:
This is the time after giving birth when physical strength becomes important. The manual explores the significance of specific exercises that support general healing, improve pelvic floor health, and help regain core strength. Resilient moms get through this stage by doing postpartum exercise

regimens tailored to their own requirements. Strengthening throughout the postpartum phase of recovery is a reflection of the mother's innate flexibility and determination.

Taking Care of Your Toddler: Physical Power in Motion

When kids reach the toddler stage, moms have to navigate a world of endless energy and nonstop movement. The manual examines how moms use their physical strength to meet the responsibilities of raising a toddler. Mothers demonstrate a dynamic physical resilience through their power and agility, whether they are rushing after little children or engaging in recreational activities. The toddler years are a time when the ever-resilient mother enthusiastically welcomes physical interaction.

Parenting's Balancing Act: The Power of Multitasking

The manual explores the multitasking prowess that moms exhibit when raising their children. Managing a multitude of duties, ranging from domestic tasks to meeting the needs of numerous children, mothers demonstrate resilience and flexibility. The physical strain of parenting becomes evidence of the resilient mother's capacity to handle challenging situations with poise and fortitude.

Fit During the School Years – Maintaining Physical Health:

The manual examines how women maintain their physical well-being through exercising when their kids get older and start school. Mothers continue to place a high value on fitness as a way to improve their own and their families' health by participating in sports, bicycling, and outdoor experiences. The unwavering dedication to physical prowess is a reflection of the mother's continuing resilience.

Adolescent Obstacles: Using Physical Power to Adjust to Change

The manual explores how moms modify their physical strength to deal with the shifting dynamics during the adolescent years, which provide particular obstacles. Mothers exhibit resilience and flexibility by engaging in physical activities with their teenagers, encouraging their participation in sports, and taking on new fitness challenges. An ever-resilient mother's ability to modify her physical strength to fit her teen's changing requirements becomes her defining characteristic.

Empty Nest Fitness: Rediscovering Personal Strength: Entering the empty nest era marks a return to one's own strength. The manual looks at how moms pursue fitness objectives that correspond with their own interests and aspirations. Mothers can take advantage of the empty nest time to celebrate and rediscover their unique physical strength through new workout routines and solitary experiences. This stage illustrates the ability to adapt to change and draw strength from newly discovered independence.

The Menopause and the Wisdom of Physical Wellbeing: The menopause is a time when physical well-being expands. During this moment of transition, the guide explores the knowledge that mothers bring to their approach to fitness. Making time for activities that promote cardiovascular health, bone health, and general vigor becomes essential. Mothers demonstrate resilience when they modify their exercise regimens to accommodate the changes that menopause brings about, embracing physical wellness with courage and wisdom.

The Legacy of Physical Resilience: Aging Gracefully: This tutorial delves into the idea of how moms maintain their physical resilience as they age. Mothers move through their golden years with elegance and strength, prioritizing joint health, balance, and flexibility in their activities. Growing older serves as a monument to the physical toughness that moms have left behind, providing inspiration for upcoming generations with the strength that characterizes their path.

The Significance of Holistic wellbeing:

The idea of holistic wellbeing is emphasized frequently throughout this guide. The ever-resilient mother understands the connection between mental, emotional, and spiritual health and physical strength. Maintaining emotional well-being, managing stress, and practicing mindfulness are all essential to the lifetime development of physical resilience. A complete approach that is in line with the dynamic nature of the maternity journey is reflected in holistic wellbeing.

The Ever-Resilient thinking:

In order to maintain physical strength, the handbook emphasizes the importance of an ever-resilient thinking. Mothers possess an enduring physical resilience due in part to their mental fortitude, endurance, and positive perspective. What gives the ever-resilient mother her physical strength is her capacity to handle obstacles with resilience, adjust to changing circumstances, and retain a forward-looking perspective.

Leaving a Legacy and Motivating Upcoming Generations:

Beyond the personal experience of the incredibly strong mother, physical resilience leaves a legacy. The guide looks at how moms set an example for future generations by modeling physical prowess, flexibility, and overall well-being. Mothers who live up to these values leave a legacy that honors the resilience of female and provides a strong role model for daughters, grandchildren, and future generations.

In conclusion, The Ever-Resilient Mother: A Lifetime of Physical Strength:

As a monument to ongoing physical resilience, *"The Ever-Resilient Mother - A Lifetime of Physical Strength"*

concludes by celebrating the maternal journey. Mothers are strong beyond their physical form, from the strength deposited during pregnancy to the flexibility shown throughout the phases of motherhood. The mother who never fails perseveres in the face of difficulty, welcomes change, and maintains her physical health with a mentality that personifies strength.

The book acknowledges that developing physical strength is a dynamic, all-encompassing journey rather than just a collection of exercises. The very essence of motherhood is a statement of resilience, adaptation, and a dedication to well-being that is constantly changing. The mother, who has demonstrated unwavering resilience throughout her life, never fails to encourage, motivate, and offer an example of persevering physical strength.